No More Brain Fog

Why You Might Be Struggling With Head Fogginess & How To Beat It

Kieron Spencer

Table of Contents

Introduction

"Due to intense brain fog, all of my thoughts have been grounded until further notice."
— Anonymous

Some days my brain would feel like an airplane ready to take off, only to be put on hold by a perpetual fog that made it difficult for my thoughts to see where they were going.

Even if I tried to plan ahead, any thoughts I'd send that far would soon disappear like a stain of breath upon a mirror. I knew I was usually a sharp person, but everything felt numb. Even the simplest tasks began to take extra energy that made my days feel like they were ready to crash down and overwhelm me.

I did not know why I felt this way, but as luck would have it I began making just enough changes in the right direction to start pulling myself out of the clouds. It was only later that I realized the term "brain fog" is a real collection of medical symptoms that many people around the world battle with each and every day. This book is here to help share what I've learned since then, in the hope that it'll help you regain the clarity you once had.

If you struggle to remember a time of clarity, do not fret. It is still my task to help you reach it.

Brain fog is a frustrating mental state that often leaves a person feeling stuck in a rut, paralyzed with fatigue so that we wind up wasting hours of our time on nothing in particular. This can happen during work, but it can also strike us at home while trying to cook, relax, or perform some housekeeping.

The end result? Not only does our work drag out and we become unproductive, but we also fail to relax in a meaningful way during our spare time. Stress increases, happiness decreases, and we're left feeling disconnected or even trapped.

However, life does not need to be lived this way. Brain fog feels insurmountable by nature, but the truth is that its underlying causes are actually really simple. Brain fog isn't an incurable disease, but is rather a symptom of complications or oversights that we have in our hormones, habits, and lifestyles.

This means that curing brain fog is a matter of self-awareness. When you're more aware of what you're doing, or what your body is battling, the better you'll be able to take care of yourself and free yourself from numbness.

This book is here to help you achieve that, so that you can give yourself the support you need to feel at your sharpest.

Although I'm not a medical professional, my struggles with brain fog have led me to this point. It makes sense to me that, if I were to write a book about anything, it'd be about helping others escape the kind of mental space I felt stuck in for years.

I will not take what I've experienced for granted: this book isn't meant to be anecdotal. Therefore, I've researched medically reviewed articles to help add depth and empirical information to what I've learned from my own experiences.

I will also do my best to write in short, clear sentences. It doesn't matter how smart you are. I know how difficult it can be to engage with long-winded text. Especially if you only have time to read at the end of the day, when you're at your foggiest.

It's my intention to keep things concise so that the information within remains digestible to you, no matter how tired you may be.

By the end of this book, you can expect to be armed with a wide variety of methods for tackling brain fog. This will not only allow you to be more productive at your job, but it will also allow you to lead a fuller life overall.

After all, it's easier to appreciate a sunset, make something beautiful, or get immersed in a game when you still have some real energy to spare for yourself. It's difficult to properly recuperate when you're always feeling completely drained.

No matter how hard you are working right now, or no matter what stresses you're dealing with, life does not need to beat you down into feeling numb.

Reclaim your brain.

Turn the page.

Lift the fog.

Start living the world with a fresh mind once again.

Chapter 1:

Understanding Brain Fog

Defining Brain Fog

B rain fog, as awful as it feels, is not its own disease. Instead, it is a symptom of any number of imbalances, both psychological and physiological.

This means some people will be able to easily treat their brain fog with only a few minor changes to their lifestyle and daily routine, while others will need to put in more effort to achieve clarity. This is normal. It should not be expected that you'll feel perfect overnight.

Because lifestyle depends on what you do consistently, it also means brain fog won't be dispelled by trying to make massive changes all in one go. Rather, it's made by incorporating small changes one at a time. Take care to patiently integrate each healthier habit into your life, then solidify it before moving on to the next.

This chapter is dedicated to exploring the most common causes of brain fog. Although you might already have an idea on what is causing your personal fog, there may be additional causes that you weren't expecting. If so, being aware of them will help you address your personal needs on a deeper level.

However, if at any point you spot a cause that you strongly identify with, please feel free to skip to one of its corresponding treatments in the following chapter. Just remember to come back here afterwards to continue your learning.

Something you'll soon notice is that, because brain fog is typically just a symptom of a larger issue, treating it will involve addressing the underlying issue that is causing it.

It's like putting out a fire. You don't aim for the flames, you aim for the fuel that's feeding the flames. Likewise, as with any other form of medicine, to better alleviate the symptom, we need to tackle the cause.

Brain fog, as a symptom, can be expressed in a variety of ways:

- Feeling easily disorganized
- Irrational fears around getting yourself organized
- Procrastinating, even when you're fully aware that doing so will hurt you
- Confusion
- Bumping into things that you should've easily noticed
- Taking hours to perform even small, simple jobs
- Failing to operate a door correctly

- Memory issues
- Easily losing your train of thought, especially after a minor interruption
- Reduced ability to concentrate and focus
- Difficulty in expressing your thoughts accurately (even if you're not especially eloquent, brain fog can make you less so)

These signs of brain fog are often stigmatized as stupidity or laziness, but that's not necessarily the truth at all. These signs can just as often mean you've been working very hard, or have been under a lot of long-term pressure, and that you now need some rest and support.

Let's look at the text below to see why that may be.

Psychological Causes of Brain Fog

Please note that all of the causes below are potential. While it's not uncommon for a person to be afflicted by several of these causes when they're suffering brain fog, you won't necessarily be suffering from all of them at once.

Sometimes, you may only be suffering from one or two.

Stress

Technically, stress can be physiological too, but here we'll explore its psychological impact. Stress is a result of our fight-or-flight response, which we evolved in order to survive high-risk situations like sudden encounters with a predator. It's a great cue to have in the wild, and it becomes even better in that context as we practice helpful behaviors in response to rising stress, such as quickly fleeing, dashing into cover to hide, or preparing our bodies for a physical action.

However, this stress response is not so useful in school or the office. You can't really hide from paperwork, you can't run from your assignments, and it's really difficult to punch a PowerPoint presentation. The natural actions that help resolve our feelings of stress simply don't come naturally at all in our modern daily lives.

Short-term stress isn't a bad thing, and can even be helpful during emergencies. However, if your stress levels become ongoing, so that you're fretting constantly about anything or everything, then brain fog can set in easily.

Ongoing stress can trigger psychological fatigue as cortisol levels build up and begin to wear your body out. While cortisol can strengthen you for a short time, your body and mind simply aren't designed to operate at that level for long periods of time, and as a result you begin to lose focus, and you find it harder to reason or think as you become drained.

Stress is one of the most insidious psychological causes since it can lead to depression and anxiety, as well as make it difficult to achieve a restful sleep.

Anxiety

Anxiety is a feeling defined by thoughts that leave you worried. Anxiety is usually not too difficult to overcome on its own but, when backed by continuous stress, it can become a chronic disorder.

Once anxiety is a disorder, the worried thoughts it throws at you become invasive in nature. They begin to distract you away from the task you're currently trying to achieve, slowly building into a crescendo of alarm yelling, "It's a threat! It's a threat! Drop what you're doing and run!"

But of course it's not a threat, and generally speaking there's nowhere to run that would genuinely help. Some people are lucky, and manage to relax when they realize there is no threat. Others aren't so lucky and, upon realizing there's nowhere to run, their anxiety ramps up as they begin to overthink and dwell in the endless possibilities.

We'll cover more in-depth treatment later but, for the time being, try to take the edge off by focusing on the fact that there is no immediate threat, rather than on the fact that there is no place to run. You do not need to run or hide. You are completely fine. Your work won't eat you.

It's important to do whatever you can to loosen the grip your anxiety has on you, and a little humor and positive focus like you see above can be a good place to start.

But is it really that important?

Well, imagine your brain as a bio-computer, with every thought and emotion you have as a task that takes up some of your RAM. Chronic anxiety is like that one annoying task that takes up almost all of your RAM without seeming to do much, slowing the rest of your processes down. It's like an unsolicited computer update that never ends, and never materializes in any improvements.

Due to its nature of introducing invasive thoughts, anxiety can encourage overthinking: as you try to accomplish your task despite your RAM being chewed up, your anxiety may find new things to worry about even within the task you're trying to focus on.

Have you ever tried to fill out a tax form, or meet the requirements of a brief or assignment, only to constantly second-guess yourself?

Are you wondering what they really meant by the requirements they listed?

Wondering what is good enough?

Wondering if you should go back and try to redo something you've already gone over?

Wondering if your redo actually is an improved take, or if the old way was better and that maybe you should change it back?

This is one of the forms that anxious brain fog can take. It buries you in your own doubts, making it difficult to see through to what's actually important to you.

Social anxiety falls under this as well, in that it makes us constantly second guess how we're coming across. It encourages us to get worked up over the subtext behind the words of others.

A classic example of this is when a person you admire says your work was fine, and they really meant that it was fine, or even nice. But because of anxiety, you start second-guessing the subtext, wondering if they're just damning you with faint praise, even if in reality they really did like what you did, and are simply being reserved.

Anxiety is exhausting. It puts us in conflict with our own thoughts and quickly leaves us indecisive and confused. If indecisiveness or confusion are the chief ways you experience brain fog, you'll likely benefit from tackling your anxiety and its underlying stressors first.

Depression

The cause for depression isn't always obvious. Sometimes it is born from ongoing stress and anxiety. Sometimes it is a result of past trauma or unresolved difficulties.

Depression contributes to brain fog by triggering a host of behavioral changes that become habitual if the depression goes on for long enough. Depression encourages irregular sleep patterns, less thoughtful eating, and anxiety.

It also leads to numbness, and can create a strong negativity bias in the brain., You can still feel as if things are hopeless or futile, even if you're living a life that others would kill for.

It's important to note that depression can come about as the result of pregnancy, or within the first month after child-birth. This is because depression can be caused by hormonal shifts, which we'll discuss a little later on.

Depression can lead to brain fog for two main reasons:

- It encourages behaviors that isolate you from potential support, and can make it difficult to keep to the habits that would normally keep brain fog at bay.

- It encourages you to focus on your grief or on past mistakes when you're trying to get on with other things. It encourages you to ruminate on the worst moments in your life, subtly replacing constructive introspection with self-destructive and overly harsh negative self-talk.
- The effect of this is similar to anxiety, but with less emphasis on stress and more on despair.

Stepping out of depression takes even more patience with yourself than stepping out of brain fog in general. You need to be willing to rebuild healthy behaviors, and stay in touch with supportive friends, while being willing to change old habits that aren't helping you.

Depression commonly hits you in your teens, and according to reported data in the US there's a 5-7% chance that you'll struggle with it during any given year (Goldman, 2019). For the gamers out there, that's about the same probability as rolling a Natural 1 on your d20 die. And, statistically speaking, you're rolling once per year.

In more human terms, the probability may be higher, as cultural norms often discourage honest reports of emotional turmoil. Be open with yourself.

Common symptoms of depression include:

- Working without a break, or always finding something "productive" to be busy with even when you need a rest, even if this "productivity" means letting down or neglecting loved ones.
- Struggling to stay on top of responsibilities (both expected and self-imposed).

- Inescapable feelings of guilt, or that you're not good enough.
- Mounting huge expectations on yourself, which will increase your feeling of worthlessness when you fail to meet them, no matter how unreasonable those expectations might be.
- Being controlling in your relationships.
- Trying to stay away from social situations with your loved ones.
- Refusing to see close family or friends as loved ones.
- Irritability and mood swings.
- Sleep issues.

If you're experiencing any of the above alongside your brain fog, depression may be the culprit behind your confusion. This book will help you be resilient in the face of depression, so that it will not keep you from clearing your mind and regaining yourself.

Listlessness

Listlessness can be thought of as a subset of depression. I've listed it separately, however, as it is specifically a cause for the kind of brain fog that stops us from feeling meaningful passion for life, or from taking joy in what we do. Listlessness can be a particular bugbear because finding things you genuinely enjoy can be a great way to start breaking out of brain fog.

This means that, if listlessness adds itself to one of your other causes of fogginess, then it becomes harder for you to break out. This can be immensely frustrating but, like with all other causes, relief is achievable.

Conquering listlessness requires that you not only be patient with yourself, like you would with other forms of grief and depression, but it also requires that you're willing to get to know yourself again.

Our passions normally form when we encounter a person, hobby, or activity that meets some unspoken need of ours. However, we are not static. While some of our passions stick for a lifetime, others are only needed to help address a specific part of our growth before they cool down.

When we have been relying on these passions to give our time meaning, we can be left lost and confused, not really sure where to go or what to do next once they've cooled.

Physiological Causes of Brain Fog

Just like with the psychological causes, you might not be dealing with all the physiological causes at once. However, just as before, you will see that some causes tie into others.

Unhealthy Eating Habits

Unhealthy eating habits are one of the most common physiological causes of brain fog. Your brain may be full of mental power, but it's a physical organ just like any other part of your body, with physical demands and needs.

When the physical nutrition you feed yourself is lacking in some way, your brain suffers for it, and it gets stuck in a state of fog as a result. In the context of brain fog, there are several common forms that unhealthy eating habits can take.

Lack of Hydration

Poor hydration is one of the most common diet-related reasons for brain fog, but it's also one of the easiest to resolve. Up to 75% of your brain consists of water. This water is needed for its comfort, padding, protection, and even helps keep your brain cells clean and happy.

Your cells must produce energy for themselves constantly to stay alive. Without water, the waste generated from this process cannot be cleared out, and your mind will soon be stewing in a nasty miasma.

Because of the high water demand that all of your vital organs require, even a 1-2% drop in your hydration levels can cause brain fog to manifest and develop.

To help improve hydration, there are several things you can already start to do:

- When thirsty, stick to water. Juice isn't as good at hydration, and carbonated drinks aren't that effective either. Ounce for ounce, nothing is as hydrating as fresh water.
- Start your morning with a glass of water, and have another glass at breakfast, lunch, and dinner.
- Have a glass of water whenever you feel tired, foggy, or frustrated.
- Keep a reusable bottle with you that you can fill up at a public tap or drinking fountain. Take a small sip from this bottle whenever your mouth feels dry.
- When at work, have about one cup of water every hour.

- Buy yourself a water bottle with time or measurement markers on the outside to help you consume a healthy amount of water throughout the day.

This will already help your mind improve, and will make it easier for you to stay on track when we get to more in-depth treatments.

Sugar Imbalances

Brain fog easily crops up when our blood sugar is out of whack. Sugar levels that are too low, too high, or consistently inconsistent will make it harder for you to think, as your body's energy reserve will constantly feel like it's fluctuating, and this will drastically wear you out.

High levels of blood sugar can damage your blood vessels, making it harder for your body to carry blood and oxygen optimally. It can also lead to excessive serotonin. Generally serotonin is a good thing that makes you feel happy, but when it's achieved through excess blood sugar it can lead to inflammation in your brain, causing your brain fog.

Low blood sugar, meanwhile, causes fogginess because your brain simply isn't receiving enough energy to compute quickly.

Sugar imbalances are a common source of brain fog for those with diabetes, as dosing your insulin too high for the food you're eating can easily lead to low blood sugar, while dosing it too low can lead to high blood sugar. It's highly likely you'll need professional medical advice to be completely free of brain fog in this case.

For those who don't have diabetes, sugar imbalances are easier to address: stick to foods that slowly release consistent amounts of energy throughout the day, such as low-GI carbohydrates as well as fruits, vegetables, and meats with minimal processing.

What is GI, you ask? It's a food's glycemic index. The higher it is, the faster it releases energy into your bloodstream... and the faster that energy will burn away. Even if you aren't burning it on anything in particular. This can leave you feeling randomly tired at bad times.

Highly processed foods and high-GI carbs can cause quick energy spikes. These spikes are situationally useful for some athletes, but for most people it just leads to cravings that trap them in a state of sugar imbalance and brain fog.

The pattern looks something like this:

1. Feel foggy due to low sugar.
2. Eat high-sugar food.
3. Feel great for a few minutes.
4. Blood sugar massively spikes.
5. Feel foggy due to high sugar.
6. Blood sugar levels dip.
7. Repeat from step 1.

Breaking this pattern can already make a world of difference if your fog is sugar-related. Note that you only need to worry about GI when it comes to carbs like bread, rice, potatoes, or pasta. In other food groups, aiming for lower GI all the time can end up cutting you off from important nutrients, and that exchange usually isn't worth it.

Nutrient Imbalances & Vitamin Deficiencies

Nutrient imbalances are relatively complex, and your diet will likely indicate what nutrients you're short on.

For instance, pure vegans are likely to have Vitamin B-12 deficiencies, which can cause brain fog. On the flip side, those who choose to primarily exist as carnivores often miss out on important cognition-boosting foods found among fruits and vegetables.

Current research suggests that about half your daily food consumption should consist of fruit & veg, slightly more than one quarter should consist of grains, and slightly less than one quarter should consist of protein. Grains can include cereals, as well as peanuts, beans, and other legumes.

The protein can be plant or animal-based, but plant-based will mean watching out for your B-12 levels, as it's the one nutrient you don't naturally find in plants. The vegetables you eat should be consumed in variety such as potatoes, carrots, broccoli-types, leafy-types, bell peppers, and more. This ensures you're receiving a good general balance of all your nutrients.

You can roast or add spices to your food without much trouble, though deep-frying isn't recommended since you'll be trading nutrients for calories and blood sugar imbalances.

Ignoring Allergies & Food Sensitivities

For some people, it's obvious that they have an allergy to certain food on account of needing immediate first aid or hospitalization. However, just because your reactions aren't as extreme doesn't mean that you aren't allergic or intolerant to specific foods.

Allergies can be mild, and temporary brain fog is one of the most common results of eating a food that you're mildly intolerant towards.

Among the most common foods that people are allergic to, peanuts and dairy products are often some of the most fog-inducing. Aspartame, which is a common artificial sweetener, is another. This is why diet sodas give some people symptoms similar to blood sugar dips even if their sugar levels are technically fine.

Another additive you may have sensitivity towards is monosodium glutamate. Normally it's quite a harmless salt additive, but it's in so many foods that, if you're allergic to it, it's really no wonder that you're in a perpetual fog. It's commonly added to cheeses, and even to some fruits and vegetables. Be sure to read ingredient labels on the food you buy!

Other foods that people are commonly sensitive to include:

- Gluten
- Wheat
- Shellfish (sometimes fish in general)
- Lectins (until peeled or boiled)

I, personally, am sensitive to fructose. You might not be, and it isn't necessarily a good idea to cut foods out purely on suspicion, as many of the above types are part of foods that have good nutritional properties.

Family history can inform whether you may have specific food sensitivities, and you can test things yourself by noting how you feel a few hours or days after you eat certain foods, or how you feel when you eliminate a specific food from your diet for a few weeks. The FODMAP diet, described later, is another method for weeding out foods you're sensitive to.

However, nothing beats a qualified allergist, who is able to do blood tests and skin tests, as well as more organized food elimination examinations.

Overall

As you can see, diet has a huge impact on your brain fog, on multiple levels! If you're battling with stress and don't know where to turn, sometimes it helps to start by changing your diet. Reduce you sugar intake, and choose to eat healthier options. As you'll see later, you don't need to spend a lot to eat healthily, but you will need to choose wisely.

Hormonal Shifts

Hormonal shifts are perfectly natural throughout life. Everyone experiences them during puberty, and the multitude of changes in your body during this time can make it difficult for you to focus at times. Stress hormones, sex hormones, and more can be beyond distracting, and lead to forming a plethora of other causes that reinforce fogginess.

Extrapolating from this, and based on common medical knowledge, both pregnancy and menopause can lead to fogginess too. Pregnancy is a time where your estrogen and progesterone levels begin to spike, which can mess with your ability to form or process memories on top of the normal effects of brain fog.

The huge drop in estrogen following menopause can also lead to poor concentration and foggy thinking until your body adjusts. Note that, in both cases, the fogginess isn't permanent, as your brain does not need those hormones to think clearly. It's just going through a time of transformation, and needs time to withdraw and adjust.

This process is not uniform, but will vary from individual to individual. Hormonal shifts don't have their own treatment in this book. It is recommended that you minimize any side-causes for your fogginess through proper sleep, exercise, diet, and more.

Some medication may also help, but it's necessary to enlist the help of a doctor or pharmacist to help you in this.

Medical Side Effects

If you have one of the following conditions, you're more likely to develop brain fog, and will need to take extra measures to clear your mind:

- Anemia—If you're anemic, you naturally carry less oxygen in your blood by default. This is typically due to a low amount of iron, folate, or B-12. You'll need to take special care to include more of those nutrients in your diet.
- Diabetes—as mentioned earlier, likes to play haywire with your sugar levels.

- Migraines—You'll need to take special care around resolving stress if you have migraines. For women, it's possible for your monthly cycle to induce migraines, as not everyone's body responds to their monthly hormonal shifts the same way. While puberty, pregnancy, and menopause can be waited out, menstrual migraines will need hormone therapy. Ginger, massages, and meditation can also help with migraines.
- Chronic fatigue syndrome—This is like brain fog on steroids. Stress and hormonal imbalances can be contributing factors.

You might also be getting brain fog from some of your medication. If you notice that you find it harder to think after taking a prescribed medicine, please talk to your doctor or pharmacist urgently, and do your best to either switch to a lower dose, or to switch to a medication that doesn't have fogginess as a side effect.

Side effects aren't a guarantee among those who take a medicine (as opposed to their main or intended effects), but you must speak up if you're receiving any. Your doctor cannot help you with alternative medical options unless you speak up.

Ditto for switching to a lower dose that's still positively effective for you, as not all medicines can have their dosage lowered willy-nilly without complications like withdrawal or the development of nastier bacteria. If you're taking something more serious than a dietary supplement, have a doctor help you adjust it.

A doctor will know how to lower dosages for such medicine safely.

Lack of Physical Activity

Physical activity is the natural way by which the body releases stress and reduces anxiety. A sedentary lifestyle may lead to low-burning feelings of any of the psychological causes mentioned earlier, purely because the small stresses you build up never end up feeling properly resolved, even if logic would dictate otherwise. Get active and see how you feel. This can be anything from a jog or walk around the park to a quick yoga session on your lunch break. Encourage your friends to a challenge to help you both with accountability if that is something that may drive you. Just getting up and active is a huge step in the right direction no matter the activity.

Poor Sleep

Any stereotypical college student knows how much bad sleep can interfere with clear thinking. The typical advice is to aim for eight hours of rest each night, but there's more to it than that.

For now, however, note that a solid sleep routine is one of the cornerstones of a clear, happy mind. Respect your rest, and you'll be better off for it.

As not everyone will be able to spare eight hours each night, and as there are many people who can sleep that long and still feel tired, we'll break down proper sleep hygiene in the next chapter.

The Mind-Body Connection

As you may have noticed, some of the causes rooted firmly in the mind can lead to shifts in the body. For instance, depression can lead to a lack of physical activity as your body feels fatigued. Likewise, what you do to your body will also affect your mind. For instance, performing even a little bit of physical activity can reduce stress.

Like we discussed earlier, your brain is just as physical and real as the rest of you, even though people often give it a purely mental, spiritual, or even ethereal quality. Your brain is not above your body, but is rather a part of it.

One of the most obvious ways in which this is true comes from the impact our diet has on our ability to think. We can also think of how our emotions can be felt in our bellies, such as being sick with worry, anger, shame, or feeling full with happiness, joy, and love.

This is the mind-gut connection.

Our brain is also not only affected by the hormones in our body, but can also affect the body through the signals it sends. Since the brain's role is to help the body communicate and coordinate with itself, it's only natural that it can do such things.

This is the mind-body connection.

What this means is that both your physical and mental self are in a symbiotic relationship, and you'll likely need to take care of both in order to keep a clear head. Taking care of your body, even in small manners, can help lead to a sharper mind, while neglecting your body can make it harder to find focus and motivation.

However, at the same time you cannot force yourself to get better by overworking your body. You need to be willing to listen to its signals, as well as stay in touch with your psychological needs. Overworking your body will only weaken and deter you in the long term, just like how overworking your mind can.

Because of the nature of the mind-body connection, it should also be noted that you cannot force yourself to become better by repressing your emotions. For example, the feeling of stress has a very real physical effect on your body. Have you ever felt like you were aching all over after a long day of worry, or after a period of intense grief?

This is because your stress, which you feel because of nervous electrical impulses throughout your body, is quite literally harming your muscles on a cellular level. This strain can negatively impact other parts of your body too, like your joints or even your immune system. Feelings aren't just feelings. Stress comes with its releases of various hormones. As does love. As does happiness. These hormones, in turn, can either boost, suppress, relax, or overwork various parts of your body.

When trying to conquer stress or anxiety, it's important that you don't come with the intention to suppress these feelings. Suppressing them is about as effective as picking at a pimple: sure, it'll seem to go away for the moment, but the core concern isn't being addressed, and it'll just cause you more issues down the line.

Instead, you must aim for relief. To treat brain fog, you must be willing to be firm with yourself, but also gentle. Firm in that you must be disciplined in performing the actions that'll assist you, and tenacious in getting up again and restarting if you happen to miss a few days.

But also gentle, in that you must be willing to forgive yourself for not recovering perfectly. This is a recovery process, after all. You can't shout at yourself for battling with brain fog, any more than you could shout at yourself for having a cold or flu. You must also be gentle in the sense of recognizing that harshness with yourself won't produce results here. Neither will neglecting a feeling just because you don't like it.

You must be willing to recognize your underlying causes for what they are, and address them head-on. Not by beating them until they become invisible, but rather by performing acts that are healthy and constructive for both your body and mind. Do this, and your causes will begin to fade on their own.

You can't always choose how you're feeling, or how your subconscious responds to those feelings, but you can choose how you, a conscious human being, will act on them next.

Actions that reinforce an unhealthy body or mind will only perpetuate a vicious circle where brain fog thrives. On the flip side, all it takes is a little self-care in one area to make other parts easier to tackle next.

The next chapter will deal with tackling brain fog in a myriad of ways. Start where it'll be easiest for you, and you'll gather the strength and momentum needed to address the causes you might not yet feel as prepared for.

Chapter 2:

Dispelling the Fog

Foreword: Building Habits That Last

Whenever you make a lifestyle change that improves your clarity, you may battle with making that change a sustainable part of your life. The biggest changes in our lives come from the actions we take every day, no matter how small those actions may seem.

Likewise, even a colossal action might not mean much in the long term if you don't make it a permanent part of your life. So, how do we do this?

Whenever taking on a treatment suggestion, you'll need to make it a lasting habit.

All habits have two basic components: the cue, and the response. Some will even take a little further and claim that there are three or even four components: cue, craving, response, reward. However, for our purposes two components will suffice.

When trying to form new habits, always remember the following:

- It can take anywhere from 3 to 36 weeks to form a new habit
- It can take 8 to 12 weeks for a new behavior to become automatic
- Old habits, whether good or bad, are a source of comfort: this makes them much harder to resist if you're having a bad day

For this reason, you want to make your changes small and simple to carry out. You'll also want something to wean yourself off any old habits that might get in the way of your newer, healthier ones.

For instance, if you have a habit of texting late at night until 1:00 a.m. you're going to have a difficult time trying to change that to sleeping dutifully at 10:00 p.m., especially if something unexpected happens that day.

However, you might have better luck if you instead get into bed at around 11:00 p.m. instead. Then, either read a book or write a letter out by hand, both of which could scratch that comfort itch for texting without keeping you up as long. Although your friend won't be replying to you right away, they'll probably be deeply touched to receive something hand-written from you later.

To give you another example, you're unlikely to stick to a diet if you change everything about your current eating plan all at once, and you're unlikely to cut out fast food or other fog-inducing options by willpower alone. However, if you consistently introduce one or two healthier foods each day, or even each week, you'll make the shift gradually, but naturally.

You'll also find that keeping healthy snacks prepared in your car and around the house can let you shake off the temptation. When driving past fast food outlets that you love, you won't give in to that *burger and fries,* even on bad days. In turn, you'll eat out only when it's completely your choice, rather than it just being a compulsion that sets your goals back.

As much as possible, accompany any new habits you form with something that scratches the comfort itches left by the old, while still staying in line with your goals of removing brain fog.

But, whatever you do, don't make it painful to keep on any new habits. Pain is a signal that tells your body to quit. If you're already a bodybuilder or athlete, you've likely learned how to turn pain into a motivator, but for most people it's best to focus on making the most painless changes you can first. The more fun you make your changes, the happier you'll be, and the more likely you'll stick with them and turn them into true habits in the long run.

For those of you who wept when you saw how long it takes to form a new habit, do not fret. Although it can be immensely tricky to form a new habit, there's a little trick that I like to use, and I think you will too: instead of creating a brand new habit from scratch, rather tweak a habit you already have.

Almost everything you do is a habit. Getting up in the morning when you hear your alarm clock is a habit: you get up in response to the cue of your alarm clock. How you get dressed is also a habit. Maybe you get dressed as a response to the cue of getting up.

Or maybe your response to getting up is 5-10 minutes of light exercise, and getting dressed is your response to the cue of ending your session. As you can see, habits can chain together. Chain enough together, and you get a routine.

Habits and routine allow you to make common daily decisions with greater speed. It also allows your brain to make frequent decisions without using as much energy, sort of like how your web browser might pre-load websites you visit often so that it loads faster and uses less data doing so.

This makes habits a massive energy-saving tool that can lift brain fog. The trick is to make sure the habits you entertain are still the ones that are essential for your current needs and stage of life. If they aren't, then tweak them.

Keeping your habits in line with your values and goals is vital, especially when you're afflicted with brain fog, as fogginess has a way of making us go with the flow of what you already know.

Proper Sleep

Cherishing a proper sleep is one of the most fundamental ways to resolve brain fog. On the flip side, sleep deprivation has a similar effect on your body and mind as intoxication. It slows your perceptions, reflexes, memory, problem-solving skills, and more. A tired brain simply isn't that efficient, and is more prone to all the mental causes of brain fog, like listlessness and depression.

Despite this, many people don't make suitable time to ensure a decent rest, and struggle to get themselves into bed. Even when they want to fall asleep, they find that their body is not listening to them.

There's a few ways around this, most of which are delightfully simple.

Sleep Debt, Duration, and Consistency

The first thing you should know, if you don't already, is that sleep debt is not something you can repay on a 1:1 ratio; sleeping in on weekends does not make up for being sleep deprived during the week.

To properly recover and get the most out of your sleep, you need to sync it with your circadian rhythm. This is the best time for your body to do all the rest, repair, and cleaning it needs to do while you're asleep.

Your circadian rhythm isn't fixed, but rather shifts according to your daily routine. For this reason, going to bed at the same time each night is just as important as the number of hours you sleep thereafter. Eight hours of sleep is ideal, but doesn't mean as much if you don't have a set bedtime.

So, look at your daily schedule. Get a journal to help you write your daily activities out if you need to. Then, try to set your bedtime so that you get eight or so hours of sleep. You want to be going to bed and waking up at the same time each day, especially if you're a teenager since your hormonal shifts are messing with your circadian rhythm, and consistency is key for you to regain control and reset your routine.

If you're an adult however, or if you're a teen in dire straits, you can still thrive with less sleep. Seven hours, or even six hours, can work so long as you keep to your sleep consistency religiously. Sacrificing one planned hour of sleep for the sake of more certain consistency can be worthwhile within that range, but note that shaving off too many hours could lead to even more hours wasted in brain fog the next day.

Too many of my friends tried staying up an hour or two late to finish an assignment, only to be stuck in brain fog that made them fall two to four hours behind the next day's work. This set them up for yet another late night that left them foggy again the next day. You can see how this can really throw off any routine, right?

So the first step is to be consistent, and to have a decent amount of hours in sleep. That means sleeping and waking at the same time each day, even on weekends. One day every once in a while where you break the rules is permissible, but two or more consecutive days of late sleep will delay the adjustment of your circadian rhythm, and leave you feeling tired.

A lot of people like to stay up late for social reasons, but for the workaholics out there, please note that it's never worth sacrificing consistently decent sleep for the sake of finishing an assignment early. Work consistently, sleep consistently. You'll have the energy to catch up on anything you fell behind on the next day.

Ensuring Consistency

Now, once you have your set bedtime, how can you help yourself stick to it? Again, we get back to cues and responses. The human body is wired to feel sleepier when exposed to darkness or dim light, and much more active and alert when in bright light, especially in blue light. One of the most obvious sources of blue light is the afternoon sky.

Another source would be most of your modern electronics. Cellphones, iPads, tablets, computers, all emit blue light that can keep your body in a state of alertness for hours, even if you mentally feel exhausted. It's recommended you turn off all such devices about 30 minutes to 1 hour before your intended bedtime. This will not only reduce the effects of blue light on you, but also help you stay away from the addictive apps that encourage us to stay into the late hours of the night.

As mentioned earlier, you can instead read, write, or even draw during this time as a substitute. Bedtime stories are a powerful tradition for a reason, and make a far better way to unwind before sleep.

On that note, you'll still want to dim your lights. Try to keep all lights around your house low during your last hour of uptime so that your brain has time to process that it's dark and it should start readying itself for rest. Most people find that a slightly cool room of around 60-67°F makes it easier to sleep too, as it encourages them to slow down and snuggle up under their blankets.

Aside from what has already been mentioned above, other changes you can make to ensure consistency include:

- Spending time exercising during the day, or stretching in your final hour before bed. Exercise is great for reducing stress, and less stress makes for better sleep.
- If you're going to sleep at 10:00 p.m., have your last cup of coffee before 4:00 p.m., or even 3:00 p.m. Caffeine's effects can easily last between three and seven hours, keeping you awake late at night.
- Don't use alcohol to help you fall asleep. It'll knock you out faster, but the effects of alcohol on your nervous system mean your rest won't be as impactful. Your nerve cells will be too drunk and foggy to recuperate as efficiently as they would during a normal sleep, even while you're unconscious.
- Have a warm bath or shower before bed. The drop in body temperature you'll feel when you step out makes you feel sleepy, and the warm water beforehand will help your muscles relax and unwind.
- Earplugs, blackout curtains, and eye masks are all great ways to limit sleep disruption from neighbors.
- Only use your bed for sleep, sex, and pre-bed reading. If you have too many activities taking place on your bed, your brain won't see it as a cue for sleeping.
- Unless your mouth is feeling dry, limit how much water you drink before bed, especially if you frequently find yourself getting up to use the bathroom in the middle of the night.
- During your waking or 'daylight' hours, expose yourself to sunlight as frequently as you can, or else have a UV light of some kind if you work night shifts. If you give your subconscious a clearer idea of when it is 'day' for you, it'll also have an easier time helping you sleep when

you want to go to bed and present it with the darkness of 'night'.

- If you're tossing and turning for what feels like an eternity, get out of bed and either read or stretch for a few minutes before getting back in. Light activities like this will help you settle down and burn excess energy without making you more alert and awake.

Physical Exercise for Reduced Stress

Why Exercise?

You already know that exercise can reduce stress. But why does it do so?

Moderate exercise encourages a release of endorphins throughout your body. These hormones combat another chemical in your body called cortisol; a hormone responsible for stress. The addition of these endorphins are a great physiological way of reducing stress levels in general.

Exercise also helps to minimize stress through physical awareness. For this reason, you'll want to eventually develop an exercise routine that keeps you in touch with a variety of different muscles throughout your body. By training and strengthening each partition of the body, you will feel more centered within yourself. Grounding yourself in this way not only helps with stress, but can even help counter feelings of dissociation that often come with depression.

Finally, exercise also feeds back positively into your ability to sleep properly at the end of your day. As described earlier, proper sleep does so much for your ability to think, and this can help you discover solutions to sources of stress in your life, making exercise an indirect problem-solving tool.

When it becomes a routine, it also becomes a shining example of your ability to form habits that stick, raising self-esteem and many other lasting effects.

How to Exercise

The good news is that anyone can exercise. Even if you're a total basement dweller, you still have everything you need to start taking care of your body. The most important thing is to reframe what your definition of exercise is.

A lot of people avoid it because they have painful memories of gym class, or simply believe they're no good at sports.

However, this isn't gym class.

- If you're exercising to the point that the motions become painful, you're pushing your body too hard.
- If you can laugh, shout, or sing while exercising, your exercise is currently gentle.
- If you can hum or carry a normal conversation with another person while exercising, you've hit your sweet spot. Talking loudly is a sign your exercise is a tad gentle, while keeping your sentences briefer than normal is a sign that you're straining just a tad too hard.

Of course, your body will naturally tire the longer a session goes on, and the more repetitions you do. Although the act of walking might be gentle at first, a full hike may hit your sweet spot at multiple points. Also, note this beautiful gem:

- Although gym class might have lasted an hour for you, you only need 10 minutes of cardio to start gaining the main benefits of exercise. 30 minutes if you're already fit and want to enhance the benefits further.

There's not much sense pushing your body beyond that unless you enjoy doing so. Exercise may require effort, but it's the respite you take afterwards that lets your endorphins work as best they can. It's also what lets your muscles repair and get stronger, leading to improved fitness. Too much effort without enough rest will only break your body down and exhaust you.

So, no need to go hard to impress anyone. 10-30 minutes of moderate exercise, four to five days a week is enough. Again, 10 minutes if you're used to being sedentary, and 30 minutes as your ideal goal when you're fitter. Go further only if you want to challenge yourself, or see this as a means to feel better overall.

You can exercise almost anywhere you want. The floor next to your bed is possibly the best spot if you're feeling shy, but public parks, gyms, hiking trails, and gardens are all excellent choices too.

Exercise Ideas

Almost any aerobic or cardiovascular exercise will help you to reduce stress, so you truly are spoiled for choice. If you aren't sure what to start with, take a look at some of the suggestions below.

- Dancing—Great for expressive individuals, creatives, and for people who struggle to express themselves through words. Dancing can easily be done in your own bedroom. It can also include potentially every part of your body. Avoid jerky motions, and take care to really stretch into the moves you make so that you can comfortably warm up as you move.

- Gardening—particularly the digging, trimming, and planting. Some people love growing their own herbs, fruits, and vegetables. If this is you, this is an excuse for you to spend more time connecting with that hobby.
- Swimming—Water is amazing because it offers a lot of resistance without being painful to move through. If you hate the shock of your heels hitting the ground when you run, learn to swim. The liquid will cushion your movements, while still demanding effort to navigate through it. A wonderful full-body workout.
- Cycling—Particularly popular with environmentalists, as well as in communities where cars aren't practical. Anyone can get a bike and find a local street or trail to cycle along.
- Dog walking—Works well if your dog is an energetic one, as they love going for long walks on the beach. A few laps around your residential block, or running around in a local park will get your heart racing.
- Walking and jogging—Bring more walking into your life by getting off the elevator one floor early, or parking just one block further away than necessary. If you love being around nature, a local hiking trail is a great way to walk while being in an environment you can thoroughly enjoy while breathing in the fresh air.
- Jumping jacks—A gym class staple that can easily be done in the privacy of your room.

- Stair climbing—Walking for stair-fetishists. If you're ever able to visit an empty stadium, stair-climbing feels best there. Some public monuments also have impressive but sparsely populated stairways that you can use.
- Push-ups and sit-ups—Often used to test a military recruit's basic fitness, these help with arm and core strength respectively.
- Yoga and/or Pilates—Numerous guides for these physical disciplines already exist, including books, free online guides, and even demonstration videos. These exercises may seem gentle at a glance, but can easily become a moderate full-body exercise with practice.

Mental Exercises to Lower Anxiety

Although physical exercise is beneficial, not every stress or anxiety can be resolved by running or physical exercise.

Nagging doubts and self-sabotaging thoughts are sometimes an unwelcomed part of the brain fog experience. Consider using any of the exercises below to address your anxieties.

Journaling

Journals are an incredible way to help us stay accountable to ourselves. We can use them to schedule events, plan our routines, and objectively compare our progress to what we want to achieve. If we continuously fall short, it's an indicator that we're either expecting too much of ourselves, or that we need to schedule time for extra help or training.

A journal lets us be honest with ourselves while letting us put down our thoughts in black and white, where they're easier for us to process and move on from.

All of these points make journaling great for relieving anxiety in a roundabout way, purely by virtue of helping you stay on track with what you want or need to do.

However, if you want your journaling to tackle your anxiety directly, there are two key ways to approach it:

1. Write expressively, with an emphasis on honesty, transparency, and directness towards yourself.
2. Write appreciatively, with an emphasis on gratitude for anything in your life that makes it feel even vaguely pleasant.

Either way, writing for about 15 minutes a day, five days a week, is plenty for you to gain the mental health benefits of journaling. It is expected that you might draw a total blank and write very little during your first session. However, even three sentences is a good start. Eventually, you'll be able to fill a page, and then multiple pages, should journaling become a passion that you're willing to pour more time and heart into.

When Writing Expressively

- Write quickly. It makes everything below easier to do.
- Don't worry about spelling, grammar, or even sentence structure. The important thing is unearthing thoughts and feelings that you don't normally keep near the surface. Don't let language conventions get in the way. Let it all flow.
- Don't censor yourself. Again, you want to achieve a greater insight into what you're telling yourself on an

emotional subconscious level. Ingrained beliefs around social norms or etiquette should not get in the way of that.

- You can be banal and write about the doughnut you ate, or you can write about the hardest day of your life. Either way, don't force it. Whatever you write is fine. Just let it come naturally, and don't be afraid to write out the dark or the difficult when it comes your way.
- Only stop to read what you've written at the end of your session.
- Consider how you feel about each thought or sentence you wrote down. Harsh or negative thoughts can be questioned with the words, "But is that true?"
- When reading over your thoughts later, be aware of how you feel about them. Do you agree with them? If so, why? If not, then what do you want to be telling yourself instead? How can you overcome them?

When Writing Appreciatively

- It is better to write about people than it is to write about things.
- It is better to write about traits, values, or other personal qualities than it is to write about physical attributes.
- It is perfectly valid to feel grateful for the sound of birdsong outside your window.
- It is encouraged for you to feel grateful for the growth and/ or success of a friend or loved one.
- It is normal to struggle with this form of writing at first, especially if you're in a negative mindset by default.
- Avoid being passive aggressive. Only write what you sincerely believe.

Prioritize Your Values

Knowing what's important to you encourages you to choose actions that you'll be proud of. This can significantly increase your self-esteem. Incidentally, it also makes it easier for you to say, "no" to requests that do not line up with your priorities or align with your beliefs. This can allow you to avoid being socially pressured into work or events that overwhelm you.

To discover your values, first think about your loved ones and role models. Pick around three to six people you deeply love or admire. Consider the qualities that earned this love or respect from you. These are likely high priority values for you.

Next, examine the most consistent choices you make in your life: your habits. If you had to assign a value to each habit, what would they be? Overall, what do these habits say about you? A lot of stress can come from living out values that we aren't proud of, or don't believe in. For habits that don't match up with your desired values, consider how they can be tweaked a little to better reflect what you cherish as a person.

Also ask yourself the following:

- When was I happiest? What was I doing? Who was with me?
- When did I feel most confident? What was I doing? Who supported me?
- When was I most content or satisfied? What desire was being fulfilled? Who or what made that experience meaningful?

When it comes to prioritization, it helps to write a quick two minute list. Then, whenever you see two values really close to each other, ask yourself which one you'd choose if you could only fulfill one. This'll help you shuffle your list until you've become fully aware of what you truly believe in. You'll also be aware of what choices are more likely to help you feel happy, confident, or content, beating your anxiety.

Mindfulness

Meditation will be covered in more detail in the next chapter, but mindfulness is always a great way to reduce anxiety and interrupt your brain fog. There are several ways to practice mindfulness.

- Be aware—Ask yourself if being constantly stressed or anxious is a problem you're facing. If it is, admitting it can be a powerful way to help you prioritize meaningful relaxation for yourself.
- Count—When anxiety is overwhelming, excuse yourself and find a spot to close your eyes, and count to 10 or higher. This helps when too much is happening at once, and you need a minute to process things before carrying on with your day.
- Become present—A lot of anxiety comes from concerning yourself with the past and/ or the future. Be mindful of the present by paying attention to immediate environmental sensations like how your skin feels against the air, how your clothes feel against your body, how the air smells as you breathe it in. Then, focus your mind on the sounds around you. When your thoughts feel like they're racing out of control, this helps slow

them down so that they can be more easily processed afterwards.

- Visualize—Imagine a setting, whether it's real or not, that embodies what you value most in life. A place where your brain can relax, and create scenarios it finds enjoyable or fulfilling. This positive fantasy works well as a buffer against negative fantasies conjured up by your anxieties.

Dieting

Because what you eat is so vital for both your physical and mental functioning, I'm going to address several diet choices that some have claimed to help them with their brain fog.

Please note that this is not a comprehensive dieting book. If you want more information, both the Healthline and Harvard Health websites are free to use, and do a beautiful job of expanding on each of the diets below.

Foods You Should Always Try to Include

This list is your guideline regardless of the diet you choose, as each food listed here is beyond helpful for fighting brain fog. It should only be overruled if your diet demands it, and even then only if you know for a fact that the diet you're currently using is the best for you. Consult your doctor if you have any concerns for intolerance or allergy.

The Golden Rule

- Whatever you choose to eat, space your daily dose of protein, vegetables, and grains as described in Chapter 1 (25%/50%/25%).

Brain Protection and General Health

Great brain-foods in this category include...

- Coffee—Due to its caffeine and antioxidants, coffee helps you feel more alert and protects your body and mind from wear and tear, respectively. One large cup about two hours after you wake up is sufficient. Remember to stop drinking coffee around seven hours or so before you intend to sleep.
- Oranges—One medium orange is enough for all your vitamin C needs, and vitamin C is vital for preventing brain decay. It is also rich in antioxidants that help reduce the damage that stress can cause to brain cells.
- Broccoli—A single cup fulfills your entire day's vitamin K requirements. Vitamin K is pivotal for forming a dense, cushioning fat in your brain that protects it from disturbances. This has been found to help improve memory over time.

Quicker Thinking and Better Reasoning

Great brain-foods in this category include...

- Blueberries and nuts—Both help improve memory as well as brain-cell communication, allowing you to think quicker as thoughts are transmitted throughout your brain faster. Be sure to eat plenty of either.
- Eggs—Rich in a variety of nutrients, but what stands out is vitamin B-12, which is important for making fresh

blood to oxygenate your brain. Another stand-out is choline, which is linked to improved memory.

Reduced Stress and Anxiety

Great brain-foods in this category include...

- Green tea is similar to coffee, but instead of a large amount of caffeine for alertness, it contains reduced caffeine with greater L-theanine levels. This helps your brain self-soothe while keeping it fully awake, drastically reducing stress and anxiety while keeping you aware of everything around you.
- Any foods rich in magnesium, zinc, copper, or iron. Iron deficiency is a leading cause of brain fog, and all the other nutrients listed are vital for learning, impulse control, and responsiveness.

Foods to Avoid

Here are some examples of foods to avoid while dealing with brain fog. This doesn't mean you can never consume them, only that they should be eaten as a treat, or in moderation. Not as a staple or habitual ingredient.

- Sodas, energy drinks, and even fruit juice. All of them are way too high in sugar. Stick to water, milk, or tea instead. The health benefits of fruit juice pale in comparison to actually eating fruit whole.
- White rice, or any other refined carbs. These are high glycemic index (high-GI), which is never a great thing in a carbohydrate. In large quantities, they can greatly slow your progress in escaping brain fog. Rather use

wholegrain or relatively unrefined equivalents, such as brown rice.

- Hydrogenated vegetable oils, found in margarine and a lot of pre-packaged pastries. Rather use butter, bake your own biscuits at home, and stick to unsaturated, non-hydrogenated oils instead.
- Instant noodles. Go for regular noodles instead.
- Cornflakes, especially the processed, sugar-infused kind. Rather go for plain bran flakes. Add your own sugar if you must, but at least you'll know how much you're getting in. Too much sugar at once can feel like eating a high-GI carb: a rush, then a slump.
- Although baked potatoes aren't inherently bad, you can swap them for bulgur or pasta as a lower-GI alternative if you're really battling with brain fog.

Diet Options

I really wanted to include a brief summary of some dietary options for you to look into and research to ensure you are on the right track. Below are a select few alternatives that may be of help.

The Ketogenic Diet

The Keto diet and its specific low-carb, high-fat nature means that for some it's not the best long-term health choice. Although for others, the diet can be an effective component for weight loss and certain health conditions.

In short, the Ketogenic diet relies on a state of metabolism known as ketosis, where your body adapts to burning fat (in the form of ketones) instead of glucose for fuel. To enter a state of ketosis and start producing ketones as a fuel source, you need to follow some strict guidelines. The most important of guidelines to follow is the reduction of carbohydrate intake. You will need to consume no more than 20-50 grams of carbohydrates to ensure that your body is adapting to the change and beginning to replace its fuel source. So be sure to monitor the macro-nutrient contents of each item as it can add up fast.

It may sound extreme at first but once you cut out a lot of processed foods and sugary snacks, you are left with a healthy array of food choices such as meats, seafood, eggs, cheeses, vegetables, nuts and seeds, berries, and many more. Herbs and spices are also fine. It's best to include as much variety as you can for the sake of getting all your nutrients in, as poor nutrition can easily make brain fog worse.

The Keto diet was originated to treat specific neurological disorders, but has become quite a common choice for those looking for better health. You are, of course, welcome to try it for a few weeks, or adapt it to include at least some healthy carbohydrates, and see if your fog improves.

Keto guidelines:

- Can be used to help treat diabetes
- Can be used to reduce epilepsy, even if medication hasn't helped you
- Kale, mushrooms, onions, bell peppers, broccoli, and tomatoes to name a few are all good low-to-no carb picks

that contain vitamins such as C, K, B (in the case of mushrooms), and antioxidants.

- A more sustainable and universally helpful version of the keto diet is the low-carb diet.

The Low-Carb Diet

A low-carb diet is similar to Keto, but doesn't require you to enter ketosis. The idea isn't to completely deprive your body of carbohydrates, but rather to reduce them to a healthier level.

If you're living an active lifestyle, and don't need to lose weight, this diet can include potatoes, as well as low-GI grains like brown rice, quinoa, and oats.

Good foods for this diet include:

- Fish, meat, and plenty of eggs
- Any non-starchy fruits and vegetables
- Nuts and seeds
- Dairy, fats, and vegetable oils

Foods that should be moderated or avoided while on this diet include:

- Seed and hydrogenated oils
- Any highly-processed foods with lots of added sugars or compounds
- Any premade, precooked, prepackaged food
- Any bread that isn't homemade specifically for a low carbohydrate count
- Pastries and other baked goods

Low-FODMAP Diet

A FODMAP diet is shorthand for "low FODMAP" which is an excellent choice for people who have major problems with food sensitivities. This is because a FODMAP diet aims to cut out a variety of foods known for causing a number of problems.

Foods rich in lactose, fructose, polyols, as well as oligosaccharides such as beans, wheat, rye, onions, garlic, and peanuts should be avoided for those with an intolerance to lactose or fructose for example. These intolerances may be causing many unwanted problems such as lethargy, bloating, brain fogginess, stomach cramping, etc.

Much like a keto diet, this is best reserved for people with very specific underlying causes for their brain fog. If you don't have food sensitivities or irritable bowel syndrome, you're better off with another diet as many of the FODMAPS this diet requires you to avoid are necessary for a healthy digestive system in "normal" people.

Some FODMAPs, such as garlic, are rich in compounds that improve your immune system, reduce blood pressure, help prevent the onset of dementia, and more. So, if they don't trigger bad reactions in your body, there's no reason you should avoid them. Test out some food groups to see if they have an effect on you.

A successful FODMAP diet consists of several stages:

- Restrict all foods high in FODMAPs. This includes not only wheat, legumes, onions, and garlic, but also fruit, some vegetables, grains, and even drinks. You must be strict with yourself in this stage if you want your low-FODMAP diet to succeed.

- Reintroduce ONE high-FODMAP food into your diet for three days. Write in your journal whether it made you feel better or worse. Either way, take it back out of your diet for now, and bring back a different high-FODMAP food, again for three days.
- Once you know which foods you're sensitive towards, and which ones you can tolerate, you can bring back your safe high-FODMAPs and include them in your diet as normal.

Diet guidelines:

- Black coffee, mint tea, and plain water are good low-FODMAP choices for drinks.
- Cheddar, parmesan, and feta are all grand dairy choices.
- Brown rice, oats, and quinoa are excellent ways to get the benefits of grain while still being low-FODMAP.
- Glucose, maple syrup, and sucrose are the best sugars for this diet.
- Go for eggs, nuts, and seeds instead of beans, lentils, or peas.
- Carrots, kale, and tomatoes are excellent vegetable choices. Avoid cauliflower or broccoli.
- Pick berries instead of cherries. Also go for oranges instead of apples. It turns out, an apple a day only keeps the doctor away if you don't have sensitivities.
- Pick berries instead of cherries. Also go for oranges instead of apples. It turns out, an apple a day only keeps the doctor away if you don't have sensitivities.
- While garlic is high-FODMAP, note that chives, chili, ginger, and lemongrass are not. Ginger is especially a

great substitute, since it contains a swath of impressive health benefits that make up for the loss of garlic.

- Be careful of portion sizing, as some choices may contain high FODMAP's in large quantities.

Paleo Diet

The premise of a paleo diet is that the modern Western way of eating is terrible, and that we are far better off sticking to what our ancestors are most likely to have consumed. The argument is that our bodies are not made to digest all the processed and packaged foods we're eating these days.

When you look at the Standard American Diet, it's not hard to see why proponents of the paleo diet have raised this point. The traditional food pyramid, with carbs forming the foundation, and fats and protein often discouraged, has certainly had a plethora of unintended health consequences.

A paleo diet is healthy and clean, with a focus on wholefoods. Instead of buying a pre-cut and processed vegetable mix, you'd instead buy your broccoli, carrots, and so forth whole and raw. That way, you can cook them however is best for you, knowing that nothing has been added that may be negatively affecting you.

A paleo diet recommends:

- Any meat and seafood, especially if free-range or wild-caught
- Eggs
- Whole fruit and vegetables
- Potatoes, turnips, yams, and other tubers

- Salt, herbs, and spices
- Unsaturated fats and most vegetable-based oils
- Moderated butter and cheese

A paleo diet requires you to avoid:

- Processed and added sugar
- Grains
- Legumes
- Most dairy, as well as trans fats like margarine and hydrogenated oils
- Seed, flower, or bean-based vegetable oils
- Any food that looks like it came out of a factory instead of a farm

However, this doesn't necessarily mean that fully committing to the Stone Age is the way to go. All the recommended foods are highly healthy and nutritious, but the restriction on all grains and legumes can bar you from many more healthy nutrients.

If you aren't sensitive to dairy, grains, or legumes, I see no reason for you to leave them out. Note that many of the foods the paleo diet requires you to avoid fall under high-FODMAP foods. It is true that not everyone has evolved to be able to eat these comfortably, but it's also true that many people can, and benefit from doing so.

Unless you have troubling food sensitivities, it's better to treat paleo as a foundation rather than as firm set of rules.

The Mediterranean Diet

The Mediterranean diet is based around traditional foods that people used to consume in regions neighboring the Mediterranean Sea, including Spain, Greece, and Italy to name a few. Some believe that following a Mediterranean Diet helps to improve cognitive function, memory and attentiveness. Perfect for supporting those of us with brain fog right?

Now, what does this diet recommend?

- Keeping red meat consumption to rare occasions
- Eating poultry, eggs, and dairy in moderate amounts (e.g. once a day or less)
- Letting nuts, seeds, and legumes act as a source of protein alongside plenty of seafood
- Using plenty of herbs and spices in your meals
- Eating plenty of fruits and vegetables of many colors and varieties
- Drink plenty of water
- Tea and coffee are great in moderation, as is one cup of red wine a day, for all you wine drinkers
- Avoiding processed foods like hydrogenated oils, any drinks sweetened with sugar, most processed meats such as ham slices or salami, as well as high-GI carbs

Unless you have a food sensitivity to the ingredients in this diet, this is the diet I recommend to you for dealing with brain-fog. The emphasis on a large balance of plant-based food will keep you rich in a variety of nutrients, while the recommendation for seafood lets you enjoy some of the healthier meats out there. Fish is especially high in omega-3 fatty acids and vitamin D, both of which help with keeping your heart and mind as strong as they can be. Fish also contains vitamin B-12, which you cannot get from plants.

If you want to be a full vegan or vegetarian for any reason, it's highly recommended that you fortify or supplement yourself with B-12 to avoid brain fog. The important part is picking what works for you and choosing something that you can happily stick to. It's important to note that while our food intake might not seem so impactful, the foods we nourish our body with can have lasting effects on our health and well-being.

Chapter 3:

Additional Support to Clear Your Mind

Making Meditation Meaningful

Earlier, we touched on mindfulness, where a whole bunch of short and sweet suggestions were left to help you ground yourself and feel more present in your life.

If you're struggling with any of those methods, you may benefit from first performing some meditation. This can help lay the foundation for mindfulness in your daily life, which in turn can dramatically help with your brain fog. For many people, meditation is quite simple, but it's easy to forget the little things that make it worthwhile when we're in a foggy space. Meditation isn't about forcing yourself to be calm. It's not about sitting cross-legged and going "ohmmmmm." It doesn't even have to be about you opening yourself up to anything spiritual.

At its core, meditation is about letting your thoughts and feelings flow through you freely. Paradoxically, it's also about you being the guide for those thoughts and feelings, but perhaps not in the way you'd expect.

Setting Up a Successful Meditation Session

While masters of meditation can perform their art almost anywhere, beginners will benefit from choosing a safe, quiet and comfortable space. If you're an absolute beginner, then make sure you have this space to yourself for at least 10 minutes. If you've meditated before, then you might be comfortable with 20 minutes or more.

Most people get the maximum benefits they can from having two 20 minute sessions each day, but don't let that intimidate you. 10 minutes is perfectly fine. And if you turn out to really love this method for calming and clearing your mind, there's no reason you can't go for longer either.

So, 10 minutes in a quiet space. This can be your bedroom, a park outdoors, or any other space where you feel safe and comfortable. You can meditate while standing, but you may prefer sitting, especially as a beginner. If you're sitting, you're free to use a cushion too. Try to avoid laying down, as you're at risk of falling asleep if you do, especially as a beginner. If you're wearing any shoes, watches or spectacles, it's recommended you remove them. Loose, comfortable clothing is best. Let nothing feel tight or constrictive on you.

Breathe

Once you're ready, sit down, close your eyes, and relax your entire body. Let yourself breathe. Focus your thoughts on the feeling of life entering your body through the air, and all the grime leaving as you breathe out. Deep breath in, deep breath out. In and out, in and out. Focus your awareness on your breath. Now that you're aware, let it go.

Let your body keep breathing, but do not try to control it. Just be aware. Stay aware. Through this, you're teaching yourself that it's possible to be aware of something without having to meddle in it or interfere with it. This lesson will help you stand above thoughts that may be stressing you out. So keep breathing, but don't control your breath. Simply be aware. Trust that your body will keep itself alive. Trust that it will breathe with you. As you breathe, gently scan your body. Turn your awareness to the top of your head, then the muscles in your face, then your neck, your shoulders, your chest, your arms, your legs, your feet. At each stage, let yourself be aware of any tension you feel... and release it. Let your muscles relax and release it.

Then, turn your mind back to your breath. No matter where your thoughts might take you, return to your breath. Often, while meditating, you'll feel your thoughts and feelings swirling around you, perhaps like a vortex. It feels powerful, but they can't sweep you away unless you let them. So, let them wash over you, but remain sitting, your muscles relaxed, and aware of your breath.

At several points, you may notice your thoughts have drifted away from your breath. When this happens, do not panic. This is normal. Simply bring your thoughts back to your breath, gently. And if they wander away again, bring them back again.

The ability to notice your thoughts have wandered, yet bring them back without harshness is a sign that your mindfulness is growing. It's a sign that you're reducing the hold that stress and anxiety has on you.

To help hold your thoughts in place, it can help to visualize an endless field of grass, or perhaps a bench or tree stump next to a road. Imagine your thoughts as a pet, or as a small child playing around you. When they wander off, away from your breath, simply lead them back gently.

At some points, you may also notice yourself feeling too drowsy to meditate for much longer. If this happens, then you may take direct control over your breath to breathe firmly until you feel awake again. Once you do, let go, and simply return to being aware.

Towards the end of your session, let yourself visualize a space where you are content. Imagine your loved ones as content. Imagine your colleagues as content. Imagine all as satisfied. Let yourself say, "May it be so," and then return to your breath.

When you're ready to end your session entirely, simply open your eyes.

Chapter 4:

Brain Fog Remedial Plan

With everything you now know about brain fog, you're already well equipped to handle it yourself. However, I know how it can make a person feel. For this reason, I've included a loose structure for you to follow. It can assist you in taking your first steps to leading a lifestyle that can help lift your fog.

Getting Started: Day One

Let's start with a shopping day. This is because Day One is a perfect day for picking up journals, as well as choosing groceries that match your diet of choice.

I recommend having two separate journals. One journal can be there to help you log the food you eat, and the hours where you wake up and get ready for bed. This information can give you a lot of insight into your eating and sleeping habits. If making the change you want is too daunting right now, you can use this information to make a more gradual shift towards your goals instead.

You can also use this first journal for your gratitude writing.

The second journal will then be for your expressive writing. It's important you have as much space as you need when writing expressively. If you're on a budget, you can use examination pads, exercise books, or even text documents. However, I know that I personally prefer something physical, because it engages my senses more fully and makes processing easier for me. I also know I don't want to use anything that makes my self-improvement feel like schoolwork.

Grocery Guides

If you're not sure what to get for food, here's some examples of different meals for each diet. Feel free to use any of them as either breakfast, lunch, or dinner. The lists below aren't exhaustive, but are just a springboard to help you dig into your diet of choice. As you read, you may notice some of these suggestions can fit in diets other than the one they're listed in. This is fine.

You can also experiment with adding the brain-boosting foods mentioned in the last chapter to any of the suggestions below.

Mediterranean

- Oatmeal with raisins
- Tuna salad
- Grilled lamb with lettuce and a baked potato
- Grilled or broiled salmon with brown rice and vegetables of your choice

- Grilled chicken and vegetables alongside a single baked potato
- Whole grain sandwiches with cheese and lettuce
- Eggs with grilled or roasted vegetables as well as tomatoes and onions
- Some fruit for dessert

Paleo

- Bacon and eggs, with an orange or banana as a snack afterwards
- A bun-less hamburger with fried vegetables and butter
- Butter-fried salmon and vegetables
- Baked salmon, avocado, and fried vegetables
- Ground-beef and vegetable stir-fry
- Nuts, berries, or boiled eggs as a snack. Nuts do not include peanuts, as those are legumes.

FODMAP (Restriction Stage)

- Oatmeal with walnuts and blueberries
- Spinach and feta omelet
- Salmon sashimi with a side of avocado... yes, really
- Fish tacos with corn-based tortillas (to stay low-FODMAP)
- Vegetable soup with beef chunks
- Beef stew
- Eggs and bell peppers with cheddar on top
- Popcorn, gluten-free crackers, or cheddar as a snack

Low-Carb

- Vegetable omelet
- Grilled chicken and veggies
- Pretty much any combination of meat and vegetables
- Anything egg-based for breakfast
- Blueberries and small amounts of almonds as snacks

Keto

Please remember that all the foods below are healthy. The flaw in keto for most individuals is in the total lack of carbs. What it does include are great foods for any diet with room for them:

- Pork chops with parmesan, broccoli, and lettuce
- Tomato and spinach omelet seasoned with basil
- Salmon and asparagus
- Avocado and shrimp
- Chicken salad
- Filet Mignon and asparagus
- Nuts or dark chocolate as a snack

Reminders for a Restful Sleep

When you draw near to the end of your first day, remember to apply the guidelines for a healthy sleep mentioned earlier. A good pre-bed activity at this stage is to write something in one of your journals for the first time. At the very least, write what time you got into bed, with your teeth brushed and all your electronic screens off. Stretching is a great activity to prepare for bed. Another good activity is to practice mindfulness or even meditation, but it's recommended you climb out of bed for a few minutes if you want to do that.

Another great idea is to keep a bottle of water near your bedside, but don't drink it yet. It'll be helpful the next day.

Day Two

When you wake up, the first thing you should do is drink a glass of water. If you filled your bottle the night before, you can use that instead. This can help shake off feelings of tiredness, as often what we think of as tiredness is just dehydration. You've probably gone around eight hours without a drink at this point, so it's good to get some more fluids in. A cool cup of water in the morning is the perfect complement to a restful sleep, and the two together can do a lot to help with brain fog early in your day.

If you have the luxury of time in your mornings, now is a great time to perform your 10 minutes of exercise. Other great times are in the afternoon, whether before or after lunch, as well as in the evening, either just before or just after dinner. I like to get my exercise done in the morning, even during workdays, since it feels like a warm-up for the day.

It's recommended that you pick a time that you will be able to stick to on most days, both weekdays and weekends. If you can only consistently exercise in the evening, then make that your time. Remember that to form a lasting change, it is important to make it easy for your actions to be consistent.

Carry on with your day as normal but, if you're used to highly processed, high-GI, or sugary cereals or instant mixes, consider switching to bran flakes or rolled oats as your breakfast of choice if your diet allows. This is for the sake of helping your energy levels stay consistent. Consistent energy levels help with consistent moods and a clearer mind.

Adding fruit, nuts, or jam on toast alongside your breakfast of choice is another great idea. Egg-based breakfasts also work really well. If you're leaving for work today, consider bringing along a brain-food as a snack.

Remember to drink one glass of water for each hour you spend at work. A large cup of tea or coffee in the mid-morning is also an excellent idea.

At lunch time, if you're not exercising, consider journaling or meditating after you've eaten. Spending 10 minutes to do this is well worth your time. At some workplaces, this may mean going for one snack break without much socializing, but you should still have time to unwind with friends at a later break during the day. Attempting to enter a state of mindfulness at your workplace may feel difficult, but if you're able to do so, you'll be bringing a powerful mind-state into your professional life. It can also help to relieve stress in the workplace.

If you decide to have another cup of tea or coffee, make sure it's in harmony with when you want to sleep. If your last cup will be at 4:00 p.m., make sure you're okay with potentially only getting to sleep at 11:00. I would advise against it though based on my own tolerance.

In the evening, you likely have plans to make, chores to do, and dinner to prepare. If you did not have a chance to meditate earlier, now is another great time to do so, as it'll help prime you for the domestic challenges ahead. It'll also help you focus on your most pressing issues, rather than getting stressed and bogged down in the minutiae.

When it comes to dinner, you may find yourself battling to fully transition into your chosen diet. Do not worry. If you cannot make a meal that fully conforms to your diet of choice, make a meal you're more familiar with, but with one or two of the ingredients swapped out with something from the diet you want to switch to.

Consistently making one or two swaps a week can help you transition to your new diet if you're struggling to dive right in. For a keto diet, this might mean having one more carb-free meal per day than normal. For a Mediterranean diet, this might mean swapping a steak or a beef patty for something like salmon, chicken, or hake.

As the day winds down, and you start dimming the lights in preparation for bed, remember to start powering devices down. If you've already journaled today, consider activities such as light stretching, reading, doodling, or creating a handwritten letter for someone you love.

Do not stress about the time at this stage. As long as your devices are off, and the lights are mostly dimmed or off, let your body unwind at its own pace, and close your eyes when you want the next day to come.

Day Three and Beyond

Day Three will be much like Day Two. Whether it's a workday, a holiday, or the weekend, your morning will have the same basic structure of getting up at a consistent time, getting in some hydration, and having a breakfast that'll keep you feeling good throughout the day. You then continue to carry on as you normally do, but take better care of yourself through diet, exercise, mindfulness, and expression.

Consider taking the next few weeks along the lines already established in this plan, but while it's important to keep your exercise and other activities consistent, that doesn't mean they can't be altered in any way. For instance, maybe you do 10 minutes of exercise in the morning every day, but that doesn't mean it always has to be 10 minutes of dancing, for instance. Maybe it's five minutes of jumping jacks and five minutes of running on the spot. Maybe it's three minutes of yoga, three minutes of cardio, then four minutes of weights. Also, don't be discouraged to extend this time beyond 10 minutes either. The point is that you structure yourself so that your new lifestyle choices can become habits. At no point are you intended to stifle or pigeon-hole yourself.

As these activities become second-nature to you, you should be feeling a tangible improvement in your ability to think. As a result, you may begin to feel bored, as your mind becomes energized and primed for so much more.

When that happens, here are further ideas for how to spend your time in ways that'll keep your mind feeling fresh:

- Learn formal styles of dancing or boxing online or in a class, which you can then practice at home to spice up your exercise routine.
- Listen to music. You may have already been doing this to cope with some of the underlying causes of brain fog. Even when you're in a sharper state, however, music is a great way to stimulate the brain. Seek out artists and songs you haven't heard before, and see how you feel

when you listen to them. You might even consider playing on a musical instrument by ear, if not learning how to read and play sheet music yourself.

- Start learning simple words and phrases from a language that fascinates you. This is a fun way to ease yourself into learning a new language and stimulate your brain.
- When travelling to a place you're already very familiar with, go there via a route you don't often take. This can help give you a new perspective on where you live, and on how spaces and places connect to each other.
- Building on that, try new things in other areas of life, such as playing a new game, reading a new book or even a new genre. Meaningfully new games, concepts, and ideas help give your perspective both depth and breadth.
- Take extra care to note things about the people around you. Focus on their best qualities, and include them in your gratitude journaling.

And, of course, consider gradually increasing the time you spend on fog-lifting activities, as they often bring other physical and mental health benefits when practiced for greater periods.

Of course, don't overwhelm yourself. You don't need to jump from 10 minutes in writing, exercising, and mindfulness to 30 minutes in each. Going from 10 in exercise to 15 or 20 in exercise, while leaving the rest at 10, is perfectly fine.

Remember, it is not the massive changes that have the biggest impact. Rather, it's the small changes we do consistently that shape our lives. Even when your fog has lifted, the guidelines around making habits and lifestyles that stick remain very real.

Use them well, and they'll continue to support you throughout your life.

Conclusion

B rain fog may be a numbingly nasty feeling, with an array of confusing causes, but that doesn't mean you're stuck with it forever.

Usually all it takes are a few lifestyle changes, introduced gradually, so that you can begin living the best life you can. The human body has all sorts of basic requirements, such as enough food, enough water, and enough rest. When one of those elements is out of balance, it is only natural that we'll feel foggy.

While there is much in life that we cannot easily control, we can control how to make the best use possible out of the resources at our fingertips. This can mean carrying enough liquids with you so you stay at peak hydration throughout the day.

It can mean looking at the ingredients you're using for your food, even if you eat very simply, so that you're at least getting as much nutrition as you can from your meals. It can also mean setting aside enough time to rest your bones, for the sake of your brain when you wake up the next day.

Or it could mean getting in touch with yourself again, exploring how you're feeling, exploring why you feel a certain way, and then working on pulling your scattered thoughts back so they can settle within you once again.

In the rush of daily life, continuously meeting the expectations set before us, it can be easy to forget the fundamentals. However, as much as your work or your other objectives may matter, you matter too. If you don't look after yourself, you won't be able to fulfill them as best you can.

With all the habits you're able to make now, I must ask that you never make a habit of compromising your basic support system for any reason. You have become aware of the building blocks needed to form a lifestyle that will lead to a happier brain.

Guard this support system like you'd guard a child. No one has any right to make you abandon the basic habits you need to function properly, no more than they have the right to deprive you of oxygen, which is incidentally another way to get brain fog.

You've taken steps to reclaim your brain. Now, protect it.

www.ingramcontent.com/pod-product-compliance
Lightning Source LLC
LaVergne TN
LVHW020322010725
815115LV00004B/37